Make Diabetes Vanish
Foreward

Dave Kazda, health educator, healer, aromatherapist, quantum touch healer, and all around nice guy, takes you on a guided tour into the field of healing; specifically in the reversing of Type ll diabetes, and transforming yourself into greater health.

Dave shows you the cause and effect of your eating choices, of how you attained Type ll Diabetes, and how you can get rid of Diabetes for good.

Dave is a listed expert on the world's largest self-help site, http://www.selfgrowth.com, has a health blog at http://healthrenew.blogspot.com, publishes a monthly natural health newsletter, and helps those stricken with disease, when possible, in person.

Make Diabetes Vanish

This book is dedicated to everyone with diabetes, their family and friends, and co-workers, who desires a way out of the devastating side effects associated with this health issue.

We all know someone with diabetes. You may know far more people that have it, than you realize. Diabetes, as of the year 2010. is considered by the medical system to be close to epidemic proportions. In 2010, U.S. government statistics show that 25.8 million Americans had diabetes, with those age 65 and over having nearly 27 percent of diabetes in that age group.

Those people between 20 and 65 years of age have diabetes in this age group at 11.3%, which shows us nearly 27 million people in this age group.

Diabetes is doubling in incidence at a very alarming rate. Colorado and Alaska have the lowest incidence of diabetes, and this is not because of less people. This information is listed per 100 people in a given area. States with the highest incidence include West Virginia, Mississippi, and Tennessee. Although many others are not far behind.

Please read this book with the gratefulness it is presented to you in. This information is given by the author, from his experiences and research over a 29 year time frame.

Make Diabetes Vanish

Contents

Index

Chapter 1
Diabetes, A Rapidly Growing Epidemic

Hi, and thank you for taking an interest in helping yourself, and potentially others, in getting your help back from the devastating effects of diabetes. Type ll diabetes, like nearly all diseases we acquire after birth, can be eliminated.

This book is designed to not only help you understand your current health problems, but health problems in general. What you are about to read here may cause you to re-think your relationship with the current medical system in many civilized countries, especially the U.S.A.

Diabetes is rapidly becoming one of the world's worst epidemics, according to the medical systems, and the press. Hopefully we know better than to give a lot genuine attention to the press. Like most businesses, they are in business to make money, not necessarily to tell the truth.

What I am about to do, is take you on a journey of learning; of enlightenment if you will, and teach you why you got diabetes, and why you do not have to keep it. This is exactly the reverse of what modern medicine will tell you. The methods I give you in this book, are tried, tested, proven therapies, that can help you easily to overcome diabetes.

Medical doctors will generally tell their patients that there is no known cure for diabetes. Or for any other disease either. Makes sense that they would tell you this, since they are taught by the ones who stand to profit from the doctors' practice of prescribing drugs. Doctors get approximately 90% of their eduction directly from the drug companies.

<u>Make Diabetes Vanish</u>

The drug companies have known for decades how to eliminate most disease. The problem arises due to the drug companies operating as a "for profit" business entity. If you do not have health issues, they cannot make money.

So why all the ongoing fund raising events to look for a cure for diabetes, cancer, AIDS, etc? Because they want you to *believe* cures do not exist, and that in order for the drug companies to do their research and testing to potentially find "the cure", and to produce even more drugs, that they must receive funding from you, the consumer. None of the part of searching for a cure for anything, is true.

For instance, the cause and cure for cancer was proven in the earlier 1900's by a German medical doctor who won the Nobel Prize for that discovery. Dr Otto Warburg. And yet, that information is hidden from the public. Unless you know where to find it. Once the cause of a disease is known, the cure is obvious.

Drug advertising alone each year exceeds $140 billion. A company advertises to make even more money. Typically an advertising budget is up to 25% of their gross sales. Gives somewhat of an idea of how much money is made yearly from the sales of drugs.

According to the publication, Science Daily, in 2007, two York university researchers estimate the U.S. drug companies spends approximately twice as much on promotion of drugs, as for research and development. U.S. drug companies in 2004 are estimated to have spent on drug advertising, mostly to the consumer and not the medical doctors, about $33.5 billion. Total drug company advertising in 2004 was estimated at $57.5 billion Is it really important to advertise to the public, rather than the ones prescribing the dangerous drugs? Seems completely opposite to common sense to me. The estimate for 2010 was $140 billion total advertising costs. Again......why?

Make Diabetes Vanish

The Wall Street Journal, in 2005, reported that for 2004, the sales of diabetic test strips accounted for $12 billion in sales that year. If you were in business selling those products, would you want that gravy train extinguished? Not likely......

I'm giving you this information to help you understand why your medical doctor has not told you how to get rid of this problem on your own. There is far too much money to be lost if all medical doctors were even told the truth, let alone be allowed to tell their patients the truth. The drug companies will go to any lengths to protect their profit machines, which is why sometimes, doctors end up in prison. Because the doctor believed another way was better. One that did not support drug sales.

The drug companies have their own people planted in the FDA and the upper levels of the U.S. government. You can do the research to verify this. I did. And it did not surprise me, knowing that many Congressional members can easily be bribed, and frequently are. But we won't go into any more politics just yet, although it may pop up momentarily here and there in this book.

So who am I, and why should you believe anything I have to say? I am one who has had several diseases in life, and had to learn to get rid of them, some of them just to survive. I have had diabetes, severe arthritis, cancer, migraines; been bitten by a black widow and a brown recluse, stung by a poisonous critter of unknown species, and grew up having colds, flu, and pneumonia much of my first 40 years of life. It is a massive relief to be able to get rid of all these issues. And being here to help you do the same, is a pleasure beyond most people's imagination.

<u>Make Diabetes Vanish</u>

At the end of 2010, I have over 18,000 hours of research and helping myself and others get rid of disease to draw upon. I am not afraid to speak the truth. And while the truth must be told, always remember, the truth does not always apply to everyone in the same manner.

I was told by my doctors, and the nurses involved, that I would just have to live with my "diseases". That my "diseases" would not get better, only get worse. Remember, they are taught this. They do not tell you this to keep you sick. They generally don't know any differently, and those that do, know their hands are tied by the FDA and the AMA, who do not appreciate people like me, who teach how to heal without using drugs. Drugs do not cause healing. Only symptomatic relief from some issues.

Many doctors are learning how to heal, although they must be very careful not to get caught by the FDA or the AMA, or they risk losing their license, and possibly going to prison for a crime not committed. I have met one such doctor. He had an interesting story to tell, which I do not have room here to give you, nor have I asked him if I could do so.

There are two things wrong with a doctor telling you there is no cure.. Remember, they are taught there is no cure, and yet there are scores of university studies that will prove to you otherwise. Cairo University, the University of Berlin, the University of Vienna, John Hopkins, and many more. , and there are scores of people who have healed themselves, or found the help to make it happen.

There IS a known cure for nearly every disease we acquire after birth. The drug companies know this. Again, you, and your doctor, are told otherwise to protect the drug companies profit machines.

Drugs, by the way, never cause a disease to vaporize. They cannot, for they are made of some of the same substances that cause many health problems in the first place. Chemicals and other toxic materials. Don't believe this? Check out what drugs have in there at this site: http://www.rxlist.com. I invite you to check out these ingredients on the MSDS sheets you can find online.

The drug companies will tell you that drugs are made from plant based "stuff". And that does have a ring of truth to it. The only problem is, that this is not real plant based "stuff". Plant compounds are extracted and identified, then altered into chemical form, to allow for patenting. With the patent, comes the money.

With the compound turned into toxic material for the body and mind, ensures the continuation of the drug companies profits, by manufacturing even more health problems.

Using the plant will help restore your health, while drugs only disguise the symptom, and ultimately, create more issues, often, quite aways down the road of time. Most of the reason one gets a health problem like diabetes, is because it is caused by the digestive system being overloaded, usually with toxins. Chemicals are always considered as toxins by the body. Remember what drugs are? The human body is not equipped to handle chemicals.

Here is what typically goes into a drug compound. Fluoride, or fluoridated water, propylene glycol, silicon dioxide, TSP, dyes, mercury, cadmium, and much more. We know, according to the EPA and other very reliable sources, , that the fluoride which is used here is not a healthy product. It is, in fact, very hazardous to any living creature. It has been well known by the the medical industry, that sodium fluoride used this way is hazardous.

5

And yet sodium fluoride is added into the water supply as a guise to help the teeth. Interesting then, that it was used by the Nazis in WWII as a method of causing prisoners to become docile, and that it is known to be guilty of creating tooth "mottling", which is a harmful erosion of the teeth. This is called "**dental fluorosis**".

This is information available in medical literature you can easily find online, and you can also find information on this on Wikipedia along with photos of mottled teeth. Not a pretty site.

When you buy a soda, do you think it is purified water? Not usually. When you buy orange juice, it is also very likely to be fluoridated. Always always, check your labels. If you cannot identify what something on the label is, check it out. First thing to do might be to key that word or term into google, with a phrase such as: **"what is sodium fluoride"**? Another would be to go to the **MSDS sites** on google and key it in there. Doing this may save your life.

The FDA states that a 3% death rate from a drug is "insignificant". I figured out how many people are sugject to drug induced death, if the entire U.S. were subject to a drug with a 3% death rate. The total estimated deaths: 10,500,000. Annually. From that one drug. At least one drug on the market during my research had a 4.5% death rate. It, at least, had a warning listed on the label. I don't believe it should be allowed on the market at all. To me, that is premeditated murder. Many diabetes drugs currently on the market are known to cause strokes and heart attacks.

Chapter 2
Eating Healthier

I learned through trial and error, and much research, with the earlier years of my education and no computer or internet available, the basics of how to heal. And actually, the basics are all you need. I know far more than the basics, but the basics are primarily what I am giving you here. Beyond the basics of health will require a library of books and a classroom of teachers to learn from. Health is not complicated. But there is much we can learn.

Eating healthy is something we should all be doing. The **S.A.D.**, or **S**tandard **A**merican **D**iet; or in my own terminology, it is **S.A.T.W.D.**, for **S**tandard **A**merican **T**oxic **W**aste **D**iet, is something that should be avoided whenever possible. Why? Because this is where a huge variety of health issues are born. That, and also with the pharmaceutical drug industry. And with Monsanto.

Getting your disease to go away will require a lifestyle change, although with type ll diabetes the change does not generally have to be a hard change. You could potentially, create new health with no health problems, if you simply consumed a raw foods diet. I'm going to give you a less intrusive approach. I call it less intrusive, because most Americans are not yet willing to live on just raw foods.

When I refer to eating healthy, this does not mean you must live on salads at every meal, give up packaged foods. Although I would highly recommend losing the soft drinks. They are hazardous to you, due to the sugars, due to the carbonation(causes the blood to appear as vomit), and due to the artificial sweeteners. You are putting your body's health at risk when you consume any of them.

And while eating salads at every meal is not a bad thing, it should not be the only thing either. Remember, I am not suggesting you eat only salads. The more the better for sure. The reason why salads alone, or raw foods in general, alone, is not always a good thing, is because as a rule they do not supply enough of the essential fats and fatty acids, nor enough proteins, nor vitamin B-12. Although I do not recommend red meat for any of these. Raising your eyebrows am I? Don't forget to check ingredients on salad dressings also.

The reason why I choose to leave red meat out of the diet is because red meat is highly acidic. In smaller amounts it is fine for many people. And yet Americans, because of their fast food / let's go out to eat, lifestyle habits, get meat that is generally not healthy anyway. Regardless of what the U.S.D.A. is stamping on that meat. Did I mention I used to raise cattle? I know what healthy is. Appearances indicate the U.S.D.A. does not know.

Red meat does have vitamin B-12. But.....do you get any B-12 out of the meat? Not much, if any. Why? Because B-12 is one of the vitamins destroyed by heat. B-12 must be absorbed into the body in the mouth, because the stomach acids kill that vitamin. The protein found in red meat is hard to digest. The human digests approximately 22% of the protein found in this meat. And yet, a simple food called **Chlorella**; an algae, is an awesome source of not only proteins, and very useable proteins at that, but also has a high source of vitamin B-12. Chlorella is considered by many nutritionists to be a perfect food.

Chlorella is also, unlike meat of any kind, alkaline in nature. The body requires a higher amount of alkaline(ash) foods than it does acid(ash) foods. The term "ash" simply refers to how it becomes once in the body. Lemon is an alkaline ash food. Acidic yes, but alkaline once inside you.

8

So am I telling you to live on Chlorella? No. What I am suggesting is that you do consume it for your health. Chlorella is very powerful in many respects where health is concerned. One of which was taught us by the Japanese after WW11, because those that consumed this food who lived near the cities of Hiroshima and Nagasaki, survived far longer than those who did not consume this food. It is known to help negate the effects of radiation poisoning.

Chlorella also helps detox the body, opens up the bile ducts, supplies the body with much needed nutrients that are very simple to absorb, and are not generally available in any real quality or quantity, due to the Standard American Diet. Another aspect of Chlorella, is that it has been shown to dramatically increase the helpful bacteria growing in the gut.

Antibiotics are one of the body's worst nightmares, in part because it kills the helpful bacteria. And the helpful bacteria is required for health. The harmful bacteria multiply at an average rate of twice as fast as the helpful, under ordinary circumstances.

Do a search on the internet and you can find a wealth of information on Chlorella. I am so convinced of it's benefits, I consume it every day. I buy it in bulk, then take a heaping teaspoon, mix in water, and slowly drink, holding in the mouth for sometimes up to several minutes to allow for optimal absorption of nutrients, including B-12. I buy mine from http://www.mountainroseherbs.com.

When you consume Chlorella, at least, any sizeable amount of it, you should find you have increased energy, more stamina, better skin tone, better hair quality, better eyesight. Why? Due to this product having every nutrient the body needs. They all work synergistically together, to give you health.

Foods I highly recommend **avoiding** include **anything** from fast food restaurants.

Stories and videos abound showing and proclaiming that some fast food products do not degrade, nor even mold. Is it true? I do not personally know. But do you want to jeopardize your health without validation? We already know fast food is not the best food around.

You can read an interesting article at this site: http://indianinthemachine.wordpress.com/2010/10/07/12-year-old-mcdonald%E2%80%99s-burger-shows-no-sign-of-decay/.

As a rule, nearly all restaurants use foods loaded with chemicals. Some examples include MSG, NutraSweet, Propylene Glycol, Dyes, Calcium Stearate, and much more. Nearly all food dyes currently used are nothing more than chemicals. Ever notice how some children go almost crazy when they consume Gummy Bears? It's due in large part to the dyes, sugars, and MSG.

What do you think happens to the average person who consumes chemicals on a daily, and most of the time, on a 3+ times per day diet? Does your car run well if your child were to put mudpies into the gas tank? Of course not. There is little difference here. You are, for all practical purposes, clogging the "engine" of your body when you consume foods with chemicals. Which unfortunately, includes the majority of the U.S. food supply.

Eating organically grown, or wildcrafted, is a much wiser choice in being healthy, and regaining health.

Since we are on the subject of eating healthier, the sweetener aspect may have crossed your mind by now. Since I will never advocate the use of refined sugar, for multiple reasons, including the fact that nearly all of it now is genetically modified, and that it feeds many diseases like cancer, and very noticeably harms diabetics, alternatives should be found.

For sweeteners we have several options. **Stevia** is one. Although this one is extremely sweet, and if you are not careful, your food will not taste good if you use too much. **Stevia** is far sweeter than sugar, with no adverse side effects ever recorded. This is a plant that the natives of Brazil would just take the leaves off the trees and chew on them. **Stevia** supports the pancreas.

Raw honey. Why raw? Because cooked is not worth much when it comes to health. That's a quick way to kill hummingbirds; to feed them pasteurized honey. The same would apply to you, if you consumed the amount of sugars they do. Raw honey is an excellent food, although moderation should always be observed. Organically grown honey will generally taste considerably better than non organic honey, and is loaded with nutrients, unlike sugar.

Blackstrap Molasses. This one many people have to acquire a taste for, although it is used in many recipes that most every one likes. It has a unique flavor, is known to be beneficial to diabetics, and of course, should always be organic.

Grade B Maple Syrup. I specify the grade on this one, because Grade A is sometimes processed using formaldehyde. It's not legal, but it's still done. Grade B is a good version. Although you may not want to sweeten your breakfast cereal with this.

Xylitol. This is a sweetener which originally came from birch trees. Now much of it comes from corn. This sweetener is highly beneficial to you, because it has none of the adverse side effects of refined sugar. It will not harm the teeth, but instead will slow the growth of harmful bacteria in the mouth.

Xylitol will not spike blood sugar levels. It will not cause weight gain nor candida. It is all natural, provided the source is birch trees. Corn sweeteners are never good for you.

If the Xylitol you are wanting to buy says it came from vegetables, you can be fairly well assured this is not good for you, since it is generally from corn. Even beets now are genetically modified, and we used to get a healthy beet sugar.

Corn products are nearly always, when not organically grown; genetically modified. And since we know from experience that genetically modified foods can cause health problems, and no safety testing has ever been done, that using anything non-organic in the realm of corn is not usually a wise choice.

Erythritol. This is a fermented sugar alcohol, again with no adverse side effects like refined sugars. You can find both sweeteners on this page at:
http://show.emeraldforestxylitol.com

Chapter 3
The Different Versions Of The Term Organic

Those that know me, know that I avoid harmful products in my food supply. So I read labels before I buy the product. I used to consume organically grown potato chips. There was only one company I could find that had organic potato chips. Several companies have organic corn chips. Not what I wanted. Well...the only store I knew of that carried these organic potato chips had run out. Then I came across a shopping cart of discontinued products, of a different version of the same brand, labeled organic.

The price was right, so I picked up 3 bags. After I got home, I was at my computer, and opened a bag of these chips. I almost immediately realized something wasn't right, but hadn't quite put my finger on it at that point. Suddenly I was addicted to these chips. That's what **MSG's** job is, to make you believe, and feel, you need more.

Well.....the product bag I had bought before only had 3 ingredients listed, this one just had pepper with salt added on the front. I hadn't looked at the label on the back. Within just a few minutes I had consumed ¾ of the bag of chips, and suddenly I got extremely angry. I am a calm, centered person, who rarely gets angry. My heart rate had gone up over double, to about 120 beats per minute, for over 24 hours. I couldn't sit still. I couldn't focus. Other than what I wanted to do with, and to, the heads of the FDA, for allowing this toxic material to be here in the first place.

It was just before I got out of my chair, that I looked at the ingredient list on the back of the bag. **MSG!** Not listed as such though, but it was there. Listed **under** various names as you can see on the next page. It's no wonder sometimes that people "go postal", or why there is "road rage". They may be consuming this garbage.

13

I call **MSG** garbage, because in my opinion, that is exactly what it is. It is put into the food supply to get the consumer, that would be you and I; to consume more food. In other words, the more **MSG** we consume, the more food we eat, the more money the food industry makes, and the more money the medical and drug industries make, because **MSG** is very hazardous to your health. And you, the consumer, gets overweight, or more overweight, by continuing to consume this stuff.

The FDA labels MSG as **GRAS,** or **G**enerally **R**egarded **A**s **S**afe. Ok....so my question is, if this chemical is "safe", why does it have to be hidden from public view? The only real answer is, **because it is NOT safe**. Check out this website to find out which words and terms are used to disguise MSG, and how many of them there really are: http://www.truthinlabeling.org.

A video you should not miss on this is here: http://www.youtube.com/watch?v=q-pnzj0c060Q. This is Dr Vince Bellonzi talking on the dangers of **MSG** and **NutraSweet**. Well worth watching. Another site with similar information, but in print, is Dr Janet Starr Hull's website, called: http://www.sweetpoison.com.

The FDA does not care that you are sick. That is the plan. By law, the FDA has much of their budget money coming from the drug companies. 2+2 always equals four.

Why am I giving you this information? Because you need to know. These products are nothing more, nothing less, that chemical compounds. Formulated in a laboratory. Chemicals cause health problems. Always have, and always will. And yes, they make it much more difficult to get rid of diabetes, or most any other health problem.

Getting to the subject of this chapter, on organics. What are organic foods? Are all organic foods the same? What makes them better than non-organic? Are organic foods worth the added cost?

There are several classifications of the term "**Organic**". This is what we are going to start with here. Following are the terms used, and what they mean, according to the EPA's classifications.

~ *Some Organic Ingredients*. These products contain less than 70% organic ingredients.

~ *Made With Organic*. These products will have 70-95% organic ingredients, and may have chemicals added.

~ *Organic*. These products will have 95% or more organic ingredients, and may have chemicals added.

~ *Organically Grown*. These are foods grown without using synthetic fertilizers or pesticides.

~ *100% Organic*. These products must be completely organic.

~ *Certified Organic*. These products are grown according to strict uniform standards, and the farms that grow them verified **Legitimately Certified Organic** by either independent state or private organizations.

Organic foods are not all the same. An organic farmer feeds the soil genuine nutrients, unlike a commercial farmer, who feeds the soil synthetic fertilizers, which do a less than adequate job for the plant, and ultimately, for you and I.

Different farming techniques by independent growers, utilize similar, but frequently different, soil nutrients. While the food is always better than commercially grown, both in nutrient levels and taste, it may not have the same measure of nutrients from one farm to another. Am I suggesting you seek out organic farmers and find out what they are feeding the soil? No. That would not be worth your time. Unless you are a scientist who just wanted to know.

What makes organic food better than commercially grown? Several things actually. One is, as you would have just seen, is that the nutrient levels are higher. This is very important, because nutrients are what allow the body to grow, to heal and repair itself.

Several university studies, such as one done at Rutgers, show you by their testing the difference between certain nutrients in given foods. You can find this information online. If you consume, say grapefruit, commercially grown, then decide to switch to organically grown and consume that on a regular basis for awhile, but then decide to go back to the commercial, perhaps due to cost issues, you will then find that the commercially grown now tastes like cardboard. I know. I've done this very thing. Not that I know for sure what carboard tastes like, but I can imagine. Pretty tasteless, no matter how one looks at it.

Because organic foods have little to no harmful pesticides or herbicides used in the production, they will not be harmful to the body. Some of the pesticides and herbicides used on certain crops, such as rapeseed and cottonseed oils, are extremely dangerous, more so than the normal chemicals used. Why? Because these products are not considered foods, so there is no limit on what nor how much of these chemicals can be applied. And yet, these products are in many foods, including some potato chips.

16

When the question is asked, "Are organic foods really worth the extra cost?", those that ask generally really have no idea. In answer to that question, I will give questions in return. For instance, knowing that organic foods help your health, and potentially can help you not get sick with anything, would they be worth the cost?

So what does living organically cost? If you have to buy the foods, it may be an additional $1,000 per year or more. So again, people will ask, "is it worth the cost?" Many people believe they are throwing money away when they buy foods that appear to be the same, but more expensive. 20 years ago, this was my thought process. Now my thoughts are that if I didn't do organic, I would be throwing my money away. Here's why:

Let's just suppose, that you consume commercially grown foods, and avoid organic. You now know that commercially grown has products added that are known to kill. So this sets you up for disease and other health problems. So what about organic? Well.....if there are no chemicals added.......why the question? But let's not stop there. Let's take this further.

Spending an additional $1,000 per year, per person, seems like a fair amount of money. And yet, what does a bout of cancer cost? Usually, between $25,000-$250,000. How about 2 bouts of cancer? What about dementia? This is not something that was even remotely common 100 years ago, anywhere in the world. And now it runs rampant among sometimes not even the all that old of folks. What about diabetes, which is affecting nearly as many Americans as cancer? How much does this cost? Given the cost of drugs and other medical supplies, doctors visits, hospital stays, potentially $100,000 or more in a persons life. Just for diabetes.

What about colds and flu? How about pneumonia? Due to loss of income because you are too sick, or your child is too sick, can add up substantially over a lifetime. And conceivably, even this could cost you more than consuming organic foods. Taking cold medications for colds and flu also help initiate you into the world of diabetes. Again, why? Because these are chemicals, many of which coat the cell walls. And what does this cause? Insulin to not be able to enter the cells walls.

And although this is not normally related to diabetes, did you know, that flu can nearly always be avoided, by the simple act of making sure you have enough **vitamin D** in the body? Getting vitamin D from the sun is the best method, and no, the sun does not cause cancer. How can I say this? Because this is a medically proven fact. You actually need the suns rays on your bare skin, between the hours of 10am to 2pm, for the body to create vitamin D from sun exposure.

Again, the sun does not cause cancer. So why does nearly everyone you talk to say the opposite? Because it **appears** to cause cancer. What happens is, when you are in the sun too long, the skin gets dried out. You lose vitamins, minerals, and enzymes that belong in your skin. You can get sunburnt and actually restore the skin to perfect, or near perfect condition, once you know how.   Vitamin D is critical as a cancer preventative. So obviously, the sun does not 'cause' cancers. Look up Dr Mercola on the web for this.

Vitamin D is important in diabetes, as it helps the body to utilize the insulin. But....you can overdose on supplemental D. If you supplement, you should have your blood levels checked, to be sure you are not taking too much. As I said before, gaining vitamin D from sun exposure is the best method. In the winter months I take a collodial liquid version, called **Ddrops**, from **Carlson Labs**.

Chapter 4
Foods You Want To Avoid

This chapter is dedicated solely to helping you determine what you really should not allow into your body. These are all chemicals, and all in the U.S. food supply, and in drugs, and in many vitamin tablets and capsules.

~ **Artificial Sweeteners**. These include some of what has already been listed, plus more.

**AceSulfame Potassium. This chemical apparently produces lung tumors, breast tumors, tumors of the thymus gland, several versions of leukemia, and respiratory disease. - Dr H.J. Roberts, from the book: Aspartame, Is It Safe?

**NutraSweet. Also commonly listed on labels as Aspartame, Phenylalanine, Phenylketronics. Since the patent has run out, several companies have jumped on the bandwagon, so no doubt there are new names associated with this chemical. This product was originally in the lab, designed to be a drug. It is very dangerous to your health. Irregardless of whether you see it now, or not. This was developed as an anti-ulcer drug, so every time you drink or eat a diet product with this in it, you are being drugged.

**Alitame. A derivative of Aspartame. Synthetic. Very dangerous.

**N-Phenylacetyl-Gly-Lys. This is considered in several countries to be a carcinogen, and is prohibited.

**NeoTame. Appears to be close to the original Aspartame formula, initiated due to the patent expiration on Aspartame. Because this is listed at many times sweeter than Aspartame, it stands to reason that it is that much more dangerous as well.

There are more artificial sweeteners on the market, especially in the U.S.A., largely due to corporate and governmental corruption. I defy anyone is those agencies to prove me wrong. They cannot. Sucralose by the way, is another chemical sweetener.

Consuming Trans-Fats, or Hydrogenated oils, is a crime against the body. And yet, most Americans really don't understand this. The media won't tell you. The media is controlled. I know this first hand. These fats clog the cells walls, which creates several adverse effects. For starters, it helps slow and even prevent your own insulin from entering the cells. It slows and can prevent many nutrients from entering your cells. And it slows oxygen uptake by the cells. All of which can cause the effect of diabetes, and all of which easily can cause cancer.

Margarine is a trans-fat. I'm not hip on drinking cows milk, but it is better than trans-fats. At least, raw cows milk is better. Homogenized / Pasteurized milk is questionable at best, if you can retain your health for any real length of time by consuming it. Pasteurization kills the enzymes, and many vitamins necessary for you to use the milk.

Always remember, magnesium needs to be added into the diet when consuming dairy. If you do not, your risk of health problems suck as osteoporosis and arthritis and diabetes increases dramatically. Magnesium is required by the human body to cause the uptake of calcium from milk, along with hundreds of other chemical reactions throughout the body.

Always remember to read your labels. And hopefully understand what you are reading. Seeing terms you do not recognize generally indicates that term is nothing but a chemical; a potential disease instigator about to go into your body.

<u>Make Diabetes Vanish</u>

Are you wondering why the FDA would allow all these harmful chemicals into the food supply? Are you thinking I am a quack? I understand if you do. 20 years ago, I may have thought the same thing. The FDA is required by federal law to work for the drug companies. The law first happened in 1992. It was then updated in 2007.

I had to learn the hard way, to survive my diseases. To eliminate them. To research, to use myself as a test subject, to find the truth. And to talk with FDA personnel to discover just what they have been doing all this time that they are claiming is in the public interest. It is not. They didn't readily give up the information I obtained.

Sometimes we just have to be sneaky about things, you know? The FDA is continually raiding and shutting down natural food co-ops. Those co-ops interfere with the food conglomerate and drug interests.

But I am not writing a book, at least not yet, on FDA corruption. This is on helping you get rid of your health problem. And diabetes is a major health problem. Keep on reading. The best if yet to come. But before we get there, I need you to understand that what I've taught you so far is necessary for your health. For getting rid of diabetes. For helping to prevent other issues. But it takes more than reading to prevent or cure. It takes doing. Will you do? I did.

Chapter 5
Your Thoughts Matter

You've probably heard the saying: "You are what you think". There is more truth to this than you may realize. You can quite literally think yourself sick, and think yourself healthy. However, thinking yourself sick is so much easier.

Science has shown us that our bodies have approximately 50,000,000,000 cells. All of which have the capability of producing 1.7 volts. Each. Imagine the consequences of this, if you understood how to use it. So where am I going with this? I'm glad you asked.....

It is not just your brain that thinks. Every cell of your body has intelligence, and dictates who you are. You think also, with your heart. Gregg Braden, former scientist, and Bruce Lipton, scientist, have shown us that your body's cells adapt to the environment. That environment includes your thoughts.

I'm not giving you this information on thought to tell you this is what you need to do to get rid of diabetes. You have subconscious thoughts that are going to be in the way of that happening. And this book isn't going to be long enough to help you with that aspect of life. However, because your thoughts are directly related to your health, this is something you need to know. You have probably heard about people who spontaneously healed, simply by thinking it. These are usually classified as miracles. Miracles are simply things we do not understand. These people "knew" they would heal.

<u>Make Diabetes Vanish</u>

To make things a little more precise, let's use the story of a young boy who ended up being confined to bed to die, with abdominal cancer. This little boy's father was a fighter pilot in the Navy. The little boy loved planes. So much so, that while he lay in bed every day after being confined there, he would play with his toy planes, and visualize them shooting the cancerous tumor in his abdominal area.

The next month, when he was back in the hospital for evaluation, the tumor could not be found. Doctors concluded this was a miracle. This is a true story. And there are hundreds, if not thousands more. I had found this on a medical website many years ago with my own research.

I use the power of the mind, or in my case, this is called Quantum Touch Therapy, to help heal. When I am working on someone with a serious illness, such as terminal cancer, I will educate the patient, use therapeutic quality aromatherapy, and incorporate quantum touch into the mix.

Although one time I did quantum touch by itself in remote healing. The terminal cancer patient was free of cancer within 30 days, and that patient not only could not afford to get help, but was unaware until I was done that I had done it. That patient had a very negative attitude. I knew the capability of emotional blocks. If you don't believe it, it's not likely to work.

You don't have to believe that. I just wanted to tell you. I wanted to tell you, to give a presentation of sorts, that the mind is very powerful. Far more powerful than you have probably ever considered. You see, the more positive in thought that you can be, the better your health will be. This is always true. And you must believe, with feeling, you are positive. Not just think it. Just be positive. Be happy. It makes a difference.

Chapter 6
What is Aromatherapy?

If you are not familiar with this potentially very powerful healing tool, and believe this is just for smell, you might want to be sure to read this. At least once. Bear in mind, the FDA has not endorsed any of what I am about to say here. I am not prescribing or diagnosing anything. I am simply giving you information that has been with us for millennia.

Aromatherapy, in its truly therapeutic state, can help the body and mind in ways you may not be able to even imagine. Will it get rid of your diabetes? Perhaps. That is not how I am going to teach you to get rid of it. Cairo University, on the other hand, might do just that. There are specific oils that they have used to lower blood sugars, and help eliminate type ll diabetes. What are those oils?

Fennel oil is known to have blood sugar lowering capabilities. Although it may not get or keep blood sugar in a normal range, it is known to lower it.

Dill oil is known to lower blood sugar a bit more than Fennel.

Coriander oil is known to be able to get blood sugar in a normal range.

What is unknown yet to me for sure, is how they do this. Whether it is by topical application, oral application, or inhalation. So what are the different applications applicable to, and why would I bring all this up if I don't know how to use them? Because......

Because as one great mind once said: "You cannot solve a problem with the same thinking that created it". If you have the knowledge of how to solve a problem, would you not do it, especially if the problem was with you, or someone you cared deeply about? Or course you would. Unless you are sadistic, and one can only hope this is not the case. Knowing the "why" of it all, is not always important. Knowing the results, is important.

I do know how to use essential oils, or aromatherapy, as it is called. However, not all conditions require the same methodology of treatment, and not everyone responds exactly as someone else. .

For instance, inflammation can be reduced by topical application of specific oils. Depression and migraines can be stopped by simple inhalation of specific oils or/and oil blends. PH of the bloodstream can be altered topical application, inhalation, or ingestion. Ingestion should only be done though, if you know for sure the oil is chemical free, and only if you know what to expect.

Certain essential oils like Oregano and Cinnamon are hot to the skin, so dilution with a vegetable oil would be highly recommended. Oregano is medically documented to kill all known viruses. So much for AIDS huh? Clove oil is high in phenols, an oxygenating substance. Cinnamon oil is beneficial for circulation.

If you would like to use aromatherapy for your health, I recommend the following site to buy from:

https://www.youngliving.org/thelegacy. This is a site I lease, only because I am fully aware of the quality of these products. I have found no other company that can guarantee their aromatherapy products are 100% chemical free. That, and the owner is considered to be quite possibly, the world's expert in aromatherapy. I use these oils every single day.

Because I have been taught by some of the best healers in the world, and I love to teach and help get rid of health issues, I am going to expand a little on aromatherapy. And again, remember, the FDA does not condone what I am saying. But then, I rarely condone what they say and do either. I am one who cannot be bribed.

Here are some essential oils, and the potential benefits they can offer. And at the end of this book, as a bonus, you will find how I have reversed diabetic neuropathy quickly and easily. All these applicatons are intended for topical use only, either on location or on the bottom of the feet. Both are highly beneficial to your health.

Cinnamon Bark oil. This one is anti-bacterial, anti-fungal, anti-viral, a circulatory stimulant. Again, this one should be diluted with a good quality vegetable oil. If you forget to do this ahead of time, you can still use it after application of the aromatherapy oil, and have less of a heat issue. Helps to stimulate the pancreas.

Clove oil. This one is anti-bacterial, anti-fungal, anti-viral, a hemostat. Not quite as warm to the skin as cinnamon, but you may still want to dilute. This oil is extremely high on the ORAC scale, which simply means: Oxygen Radical Absorbance Capacity. I will get into what that actually means in a minute.

Cypress oil. This one is helpful for the pancreas, and is also helpful with circulatory issues. This also has a capacity to be used like a styptic stick. In other words, if you cut yourself shaving, this will help stop the bleeding.

Coriander oil. This one is highly anti-fungal and anti-bacterial. It is also potentially one of the best for helping lower blood sugars.

Dill oil. This one is also anti-bacterial, anti-fungal, and is known to help lower blood sugars. If you notice as we go, nearly all essential oils that help lower blood sugars are also anti-fungal. Tells you something, doesn't it?

Fennel oil. This one is anti-inflammatory, anti-diabetic, anti-tumoral, and increases metabolism. Bear in mind that with these oils, and what is stated about them, that this is factual information that is not only current, but also discovered from writings as far back in some cases, as being over 6,000 years old.

Fleabane oil. Although it is rare I that I've seen this one sold by itself, the information should still be given here. This one is medically recognized as helping to stimulate the liver and pancreas, stimulate growth hormone, reduces blood pressure.

Geranium oil. This oil has been used for centuries in the regeneration of the skin and nerve endings. This oil is anti-bacterial, anti-fungal, improves blood flow, stimulates the liver and pancreas, dilates the bile ducts for liver detox, and revitalizes skin cells. Medical uses of this oil include hepatitis, fungal infections, viral infections, herpes, shingles, circulation problems. Inhalation is known to increase the spirits and balance the emotions.

Helichrysum oil. This oil is known to be anti-viral, to protect, stimulate and detox the liver, in addition to helping remove chemicals and other toxins out of the body, and helps regenerate nerves.

Juniper oil. This oil works as a digestive cleanser and stimulant, helps in purifying and detoxing the body, helps with regeneration of nerves, improves circulation through the kidneys. It also helps to keep blood sugar levels more in balance.

Lemon oil. This oil is one of my favorites. I have used it to help restore eyesight, remove grease faster than just about anything else I've ever used, and just a drop in a glass of tap water will inactive chlorine in about 60 seconds. Chlorine kills. You do not want this in your water.

Lemon oil is pressed from the rind, is known to be very powerful as an anti-bacterial agent ~ including being able to kill staph, meningococcus bacteria, pneumococcus bacteria, and diptheria bacteria very rapidly. Inhalation of this oil helps increase memory and promotes clarity of thought.

Lemongrass oil. This oil is perhaps one of the least used, and potentially one of the most needed by those who consume the Standard American Diet. This oil is known to help digestive issues, it is anti-fungal, anti-bacterial, anti-inflammatory, helps to regenerate tissues and ligaments, dilates blood vessels, improves circulation, and promotes lymphatic flow by inhalation of the oil. This also increases the blood's PH..

Oregano oil. This oil is quite probably the most powerful anti-viral product ever found. This outclasses every drug on the market in killing hazards such as ecoli, according to medical literature. Without the adverse side effects pharmaceutical drugs offer. As you saw above, this oil is a hot oil, requiring dilution.

Oregano should only be used topically, and only on the bottom of the feet for a novice, is the best place to use. Remember, when applying oils to the feet, to not put on socks and shoes for about 15 minutes, or you may have smells in your shoes you do not want. That, and putting on socks too quickly can cause oils to get between the toes due to the sweat produced with socks, which nearly always will be very uncomfortable.

Peppermint oil. This is part of a blend used by thieves in the 15th century, to protect themselves from the dead and dying, due to the black plague. **Peppermint oil** is anti-inflammatory, anti-tumoral, anti-parasitic, anti-fungal, highly regarded as a digestive stimulant. Inhalation is beneficial in stimulating the conscious mind. Something else you would NEED to know, is something I had to learn the hard way.

When applying **peppermint** it is, of course, on your hands. If you put your fingers anywhere near the eyes shortly afterwards without a dilution already on your hands, you probably will not be able to have your eyes open for up to 15 minutes. The fumes are that strong.

All therapeutic quality aromatherapy is much more powerful than the herb or food itself. And, being of a minute liquid nature, it will easily and rapidly penetrate the skin and enter every cell of the body within minutes. So remember, do not put your hands near your eyes for about 15 minutes after using **peppermint.**

Pine oil. This one is commonly adulterated and instead of pine, is often actually turpentine. So be cautious on who you get your oils from, if you choose to use them. The link I gave you earlier I have complete faith in. The owner of this company is the reason I am alive today. Because of what he taught me, and because of his products and his desire to have the best products possible. Pine is considered anti-diabetic, is hormone-like, a lymphatic stimulant, and revitalizes the body, mind and spirit. By scent, this oil is uplifting.

Wintergreen oil. This oil is similar to Birch oil. True birch, now, is hard to locate. These are both nature's aspirin. If you put a drop on your wrist and rub your wrists together, it will thin your blood in seconds, just as aspirin will. This is important, and on the next page, I will explain why.

~ Aspirin is a chemical you do not want in your body, and is sometimes tainted with things worse than chemicals. When your blood sugar rises, if you look at the blood under an electron microscope, you will see what appears to be cut glass flowing through your veins. This is the reason why diabetics lose their sight, their kidneys, their toes, and why they get diabetic neuropathy. These sugar (glass) crystals flowing through the bloodstream cut your artery walls. For this reason, I recommend using either or both of the following:

Clove oil. Applied on the bottom of the feet at least twice daily, if you have blood sugar too high. You can take this internally, however, if you do so, be forewarned that until you get used to it, you should not use more than 3 drops in a 00 capsule.

The reason for this is because **Clove oil** will begin to detox you, and you may not be able to handle the rapidness of the detox. I have been known to take 20 drops or more in a capsule up to twice daily, but I have been doing it for over a decade. It is very important due to its anti-oxidant capabilities, which is what I have referenced earlier, that I would get to in a minute.

Wintergreen oil. This is referenced later as well. But very important for high blood sugars, to help thin the blood to slow and hopefully negate many of the harmful effects of the cut glass effect of high sugar levels.

But first, let's discuss what the measure of anti-oxidants are. The term **ORAC is used to describe the capability of a food or herb to determine how effective it is in helping the body recover from hazards including high blood sugars.**

When we look at the values, foods such as carrots come in with a figure of about 200 on the **O**xygen **R**adical **A**bsorbent **C**apacity, or **ORAC**, scale; strawberries come in about 1200, raspberries about 1300, blueberries about 2400, and pomegranites at about 3000. Chinese Wolfberry, or you may know this one better as Lycium, or Goji Berry; comes in around 25,000. And yet, Clove oil comes in at over the 1,000,000 mark!   This works whether it is applied topically or taken internally. The higher the **ORAC** number, the more potent the anti-oxidant capability.

Brunswick Labs developed this scale for the USDA. Brunswick Labs told me in 2005, that they no longer allow for public viewing of the **ORAC** scale due to unethical and improper uses by some people. I have seen some of those improper uses. Many essential oils are quite high on the **ORAC** scale due to their concentrated nature. .

There are many more essential oils on the market that you may benefit from, but the ones I've given you are the ones that I feel would be most beneficial to you, if you choose to use them. It is saddening to know, that much of what you find in the marketplace in aromatherapy, is actually little more than chemical water.

If you find essential oils in clear bottles, they are guaranteed junk, regardless of what anyone has on the label. The reason for this, is that oils are subject to loss of quality with exposure to light. So for therapeutic quality, amber or cobalt colored glass is what is used. Although it too, may be used to disguise chemical water claiming to be essential oils.

I have tested most of the brands on the market, and sadly, many of them have little value. However, I'm not here to put down companies, but to help you. If the packager has truly quality oils, they will not put them in clear bottles.

Chapter 7
This Is How You Lose Diabetes

What I've given you so far will be helpful to you, should you choose to use it. If you do not, or do not believe it will and won't attempt it, please pass the book on to someone who may. Following, in this chapter, you will find how I help others, both in person and at a distance, get rid of type ll diabetes.

This method has not failed, at least so far in my experiences, in eliminating type ll diabetes. And in a short period of time. There are no adverse side effects in this methodology, only good effects. So let's get on with discovering the answers you are seeking. And bear in mind, this is not the only way of reversing diabetes, but is perhaps one of the fastest and least intrusive on the diet.

First things first. You should reduce or eliminate dairy products. If you intend to continue using dairy, it is highly recommended you use raw, and preferably organic raw milk while you still can. Rice milk or nut butter milk are good substitutes, if you can find some without chemicals. Might be better to make your own.

The FDA is on a mission to put natural farmers and producers out of business, so realize raw milk may not always be available in the general marketplace. I'm not joking here. The dairy industry has lobbyists who lobby Congress to stop the competition of the raw foods industry. This has been happening for quite a few years, and likely will for many more.

Next, you will want to be sure you completely eliminate the bad fats in your diet. Bad fats do not mean saturated fats. What this means is the trans-fats, or hydrogenated oils, and there are some normal vegetable oils that are better than others. If you leave the trans-fats in the diet, getting rid of diabetes may become close to impossible.

Saturated fat is not necessarily a bad thing. For instance, coconut oil, which has had a huge amount of negative press over the last few decades, is saturated, and is about the best oil you can use. It received all this bad press from the margarine industry lobbying Congress and the FDA, to spread the bad word about saturated fats. Of course, back when this all started, most of us had no idea there was any difference in saturated fats. Now we know there is. And margarine is dangerous for your health.

Did you know.....tI was unable to find a critter alive, short of a human, which will consume margarine? If you have a tub of margarine, stick it outside with no lid, and see how long it stays there, uneaten. Your kids getting into it while it's out there does not count.

Next, you will need to reduce or eliminate as much as possible in the refined sugars arena. In other words, if the word "sugar" is listed on a package, don't touch the package or the product inside. Refined sugar is not the main enemy here. But it is something that is not designed by the human body to handle on a regular basis. If it were, we would find plants growing wild as refined sugars. Makes sense, doesn't it?

Xylitol and Erythritol are your best options for sweetening, as far as health is concerned. Also, you can use fresh juice from pears, peaches or apples as well, although this may be a bit more costly.

There are two teas that are known to be very helpful in helping get rid of type ll diabetes. Those tea names are: **Essiac** and **Huckleberry.** Just to give a little background on these teas,

Essiac is an herbal blend known to help eliminate certain cancers. **Essiac** helps to cleanse the digestive system, and alkalinize the blood. The original version of **Essiac**, which I still use today, consists of four herbs. Those are:

~ **Slippery Elm Bark**
~ **Sheep Sorrel**
~ **Burdock Root**
~ **Rhubarb Root**

Rene Caisse, the Canadian woman who made **Essiac**(which was her name spelled backwards) famous as a cancer cure, gave us some valuable insight. She discovered that **Slippery Elm Bark** lubricates bones and joints, gathers up toxic waste material from all areas of the body, and helps remove them.

Slippery Elm Bark slows down the entry of harmful chemicals, reduces the pain of ulcers, and eventually heals them. The herb is also said to have the ability to cause the body to grow new cells to repair tissues.

****Remember though, and for once, I have to agree with the FDA; no herb, no food, no supplement, can cure you. This is not how life works. What you are doing when you consume herbs, foods, or/and supplements, is giving the body the tools to heal itself. Just like chemo appears to help some with cancer, all it is is just a tool. If the body can recover from that tool, then it may be able to heal. Sometimes though, as with chemo, the tool is more dangerous than the disease.****

Sheep Sorrel, according to Rene Caisse, could be the most active cancer fighter among all the herbs present in this old Indian brew. Rene observed that not only was Sheep Sorrel effective in attacking and breaking down tumors, it was also effective in alleviating many chronic conditions and degenerative diseases.

Burdock Root has been known for centuries to natural healers thoughout the world as a powerful blood purifier. This herb is known to improve elimination of toxic materials in the body, which then helps to relieve liver toxicity. Some Asian cultures consider **Burdock Root** to be a powerful rejuvenator and aphrodisiac.

Rhubarb Root is another powerful detoxifying herb which has been used for centuries throughout the world. **Rhubarb Root** helps cleanse the liver(this is especially important for diabetics), stimulates the gall bladder, and helps eliminate parasites.

According to the book: *The Essiac Report*, this tea is a powerful aid in being able to help eliminate various diseases in addition to cancer, including:

Multiple Sclerosis
Diabetes
Parkinsons
Chronic Fatigue Syndrome
Sleeping Disorders
Warts, and much more.

Huckleberry tea, as I said earlier, is known by many healers to help eliminate diabetes on its own. However, using either of these teas by themselves is not likely to get the job done. If you don't stop the insult to the body with the sugar, hydrogenated oils, artificial sweeteners, etc., then it is little more than adding a small bandaid to a large gash. It will help, but probably won't stop the problem.

I do not have the personal experience of getting rid of type ll diabetes using **Huckleberry tea**. But I wanted you to have the information just in case you wish to use it. I do know first hand, that **Essiac tea** does work for diabetes.

What I do know about **Huckleberry tea** from personal experience, it that it is a very powerful cleanser. The way I originally found this out, was somewhere around the year 1999, I was taking this tea to work in a Stanley Stainless Steel thermos I had just purchased for this, since I wasn't too hip on using plastic thermos bottles for hot liquids to drink.

About the 4th day into taking this tea to work, I was busy and neglected to even open the thermos. When I got home that night, I didn't take the time to clean the thermos out.

What I discovered the next morning gave me a whole new appreciation for that tea. When I opened the thermos and drained it, I found that the inside stainless coating of the liner, where the tea had been sitting, was dissolved out of the thermos.

Huckleberry tea can be in the form of tea made from twigs(my favorite), or the flowers, or the berry. The last two are a bit strong for me, which is why I prefer the twig version. I use both these teas now for general health, but generally will use **Essiac** more than **Huckleberry**, partly due to taste. For me, **Essiac** tastes better.

So, a final note on this. Remember to reduce or/and eliminate the food products specified earlier, drink your tea(s). Only one is truly necessary from my experiences, and keep your thoughts as positive as possible. Feel with your heart. Feel that you are healed. Your heart harbors the majority of your body's intelligence. Your heart knows what is true. And true for you. Before the mind does. And this is scientifically proven.

Listen to your heart. Love your heart. Love yourself. Know that you are on the path to perfect health. And in doing so, you will get there sooner. Don't just think it. Know it. Don't just believe it. Know it.

And as any good doctor would tell you, it is not wise to quit any medication cold turkey. Wean yourself off your med(s) as you notice you are doing better. The faster you can wean yourself, the faster you will heal.

Bonus
Chapter 8
Getting Rid Of Diabetic Neuropathy

The U.S. medical system's response to diabetic neuropathy, is "medicate until you amputate". Amputation should never be considered without gangrene already being in place, and even then, were it on me, I would probably not go there, knowing what I do about how to get rid of it first hand.

And this is how I do it.........Take the essential oils (therapeutic quality only) of Lemon and Peppermint, and Cypress if you wish(not a bad idea since it helps circulation), and put a few drops on location. Then massage into the skin.

One oil at a time is fine, and actually preferred by me. When I had had neuropathy years and years ago, I knew the devastating effects this could have on my life. And since I had been learning aromatherapy from a world leader in that field, Don Gary Young, of Young Living Essential Oils, I decided to use the **Lemon** and **Peppermint** on myself. After all, what did I have to lose, but a few dollars if it didn't work? It did work. So I lost nothing, and gained my feet and legs back to full health.

I knew some of the properties of these two oils, which is why I selected them. That, and intuition guides me well. **Lemon**, because it improves micro-circulation, increases cellular flexibility and strength, and is alkalizing to the blood, is almost a no-brainer when one understands what aromatherapy actually is.

Peppermint oil was more of an intuitive nudge, when I decided to use this oil. Both these oils will add oxygen into the body's cells. When we realize that the prime cause of diabetic neuropathy is a lack of oxygen to the cells, we realize any oil that will supply oxygen is fair game. And these two are not the only oils that can do this.

Peppermint oil is anti-inflammatory, cooling to the skin, relieves pain, and is part of the 4 oil blend used by a band of thieves who looted the dead and dying during the plague of the 15th century. Those thieves neither got sick nor died of the plague. This is a matter of historical record.

Cypress oil is well known to improve circulation and strengthens blood capillaries. It also discourages fluid retention. According to Jean Valnet, M.D., this oil is used medicinally(in countries other than the U.S.A.), to treat diabetes, circulatory disorders, and cancers. I have not used this one for neuropathy, but again, wanted to put it in here for a matter of record, for you, in the event you want to try another oil as well.

Things you need to know, if you are not familiar with aromatherapy.

Especially with **Peppermint oil,** never put the oil anywhere near the eyes or ears. And this included putting the hands near the eyes after applying elsewhere. The fumes are just too strong, and your eyes will potentially water so badly you cannot keep them open for quite awhile. I had to learn this the hard way. Keep your hands away from the eyes for at least 15 minutes after application with your hands.

Peppermint oil by smell, is powerful in helping memory, is purifying and stimulating to the conscious mind. It also is shown to block headache pain.

Lemon oil, like **Peppermint**, should not get near the eyes. And never get any oils into the eyes. If you do, call a doctor immediately. A natural doctor may be best to call, as they may have experience with aromatherapies.

Lemon is powerful in relieving athletes foot, is known to help eyesight when applied on the feet. Always make sure to NOT get these oils between the toes. And always be sure to not put on shoes or socks for about 15 minutes after application on the feet. If you do, the sweat glands in your feet will cause the oils potentially, to get between the toes, in which case your toes will then burn and itch throughout the day. **Lemon oil** in water is said to kill Chlorine.

The best dilution for aromatherapy is always a good quality vegetable oil. So if you do get the burn and itch between the toes, rub some olive or similar oil on top of the aromatherapy oil, and the problem will disappear much faster.

Essential oils should only be taken internally, if you are absolutely sure they are truly pure oils, and if you know a bit about the oils. They are very potent, up to 200 times more potent than the plant they came from, due to the concentrated nature of the oils. The FDA states that an oil can state "Pure", and be only 5% pure oil. Always question quality. I had to learn to do this for survival. You may have to also.

I don't know for sure now where you can find the **Huckleberry twig tea**, but no doubt you should be able to find it online. **Essiac Tea** I purchase from *Loriens Herbs and Natural Foods, in Spokane, Wa*. They stock this in bulk, so you can buy it by the ounce. Depending on your needs and wants, you may want to buy it by the pound. *Loriens* phone number is 509-456-0702. Just key into Google: *Loriens Herbs*.

One final reminder on essential oils, is that using water for dilution only hastens absorption, and increases the heat of the oil. And, certain oils, and **Lemon** is one of these, may eat plastics. So if you have it recently on your hands, and you pick up something plastic, such as a container for a drink of water, you are very likely going to leave your fingerprints permanently in that plastic container.

Again, please remember, any essential oil should never be placed near the eyes nor ears unless you know what you are doing. I have 15 years of daily use both on myself and others to draw upon, so I'm familiar with them.

That's it. It really is this simple. And.....because you have purchased this book, I am making an offer to you. If you have a desire to receive one-on-one help with a health issue, you can ask for and receive my help at no charge.

Simply email me at: knowledge_quest2002@yahoo.com. Be sure to put in the subject line: "**Health Help Request**". This part is very important. I get so many emails every day, and many are spam, that unless I know I should open it, it very likely would go into the junk or trash. I don't want to miss helping you, so please remember to put that in the subject line, if you choose to make a request.

About The Author

As a recipient of 4 diseases, from diabetes to arthritis, to migraines, to cancer, Dave Kazda had to learn how to eliminate them to help ensure his own survival.

Dave has taught health class in person, publishes a natural health newsletter by free subscription, publishes a health blog at: http://healthrenew.blogspot.com, and works one-on-one with those stricken with health problems, who find that the allopathic medical system cannot help them in the manner they choose.

Dave has dedicated his life to research, and helping others in their quests to help themselves, and those they love. Love is an extraordinarily powerful tool. And it must not be lost. It is an emotion. And we are all emotion based. Using emotion requires heart involvement, and can cause things to happen that the mind, and science, says are impossible. Although science is now catching on to this.

The responses Dave receives from those he helps is highly uplifting. He learned the "Pay it forward" concept in 1987, after being helped while stranded on the road with temperatures well into the 100's. The "Pay it forward" concept is an incredibly powerful concept that Dave incorporated into his own life, and has lived by that ever since.

The end.

Notes

Notes